Until the Streets of the Hood Flood with Green

The Story of The Electric Smoothie Lab Apothecary (TESLA)

By Kelly Curry

© 2018 Kelly Curry /Freedom Voices
Cover Art ©2016 Annie Morgan Banks
www.anniebanks.net

P.O. Box 423115, San Francisco,
California, United States 94142
www.freedomvoices.org
orders@freedomvoices.org

Distributed to the trade by:
AK Press, 370 Ryan Ave. #100, Chico, CA 95973; akpress.org

Published with the support of
Reimagine! Movements Making Media
www.reimaginerpe.org

TABLE OF CONTENTS

YOU HAVE TO MOVE NUTRITION THROUGH THE COMMUNITY 5

KETCHUP IS NOT A VEGETABLE 10

FEED THE 5,000 24

THAT WHICH IS FREE AND ABUNDANT 28

PLANTING JUSTICE 32

PAULA 35

HOW ARE YOU HEALING TODAY 49

QUIET ON THE SET 51

THE TABLE 58

INSIDE THE GREEN SMOOTHIE 62

ABOUT THE AUTHOR 65

Thanks to everybody who gives time, love, energy and vision in service to the liberation and nourishment of children everywhere, so that they may be free, happy and whole.

You know who you are.

YOU HAVE TO MOVE NUTRITION THROUGH THE COMMUNITY

About four years ago, when I was working with the historic People's Grocery in West Oakland, we were tapped by Prescott Elementary to come set up a table and talk about Food Justice at a health fair. I didn't think the kids would wanna hear about their neighborhoods being a food desert, so I brought my Vitamix and I made Green Smoothies to go along with all the bad news I had to share with them about the lack of access to living food in their community, and the reasons why.

They set us up in a cozy little corner at the edge of the fair, near the garden, behind the BBQ stand. At some point, an elder from the community approached me and whispered something that would change my life. "You used to be an organization that fed people, you moved the nutrition through the community, now you just talk about it. THIS is what you need to be doing." She pointed at the smoothie and drank it, holding out her cup for more.

I listened without judgment. Her words seared themselves into my consciousness—like directions on a map that I was eager to follow.

West Oakland is a place known to activists worldwide as a 'food desert', where you can go, walk, ride, drive for blocks and not encounter one living thing to eat, so when one week later Bikes for Life asked us to come and table at their healthy living event, I brought a little table, my Vitamix, a few pounds of bananas, some pineapples, bags and bags of greens, some ice, and set up shop.

Before I could finish prepping, a cute, hearty little boy came and stood next to me, totally interested in what I was doing.

"Whatchu gon' have at your stand?!"
"Smoothies!"
"I have diabetes, is it safe for me to drink?"
He was 8 or 9. His words sliced through my heart. If there

had been time for me to excuse myself and cry, wipe my eyes and continue my work I would have. But I had to pretend like his words didn't hurt me, and I kept it moving.

"This," I told him as I handed it to him, "is totally safe." I used less banana than usual, and threw in some extra greens. After a few sips, he stopped drinking and said he wanted to save the rest for his mom. She too had diabetes. I heard him zip away on his bike and I continued prepping. Before I had peeled my bananas and laid out the rest of my fruit, he was back. And he had a friend with him. They both wanted one, plus one more for their moms. Of course I was thrilled, because I'd not only just gotten the green light from their moms, but they had sent them back on a mission to get one of our Green Smoothies for themselves! The elder's voice came back to me. I remembered the look in her eyes when she pointed at the cup. "THIS is what you need to be doing."

By following her map, her directions, li'l homie was drinking a Green Smoothie on a street corner in West Oakland on a Saturday morning and coming back for more and bringing his people. I felt a Cosmic rush of love and joy, got goosebumps. The beautiful bright expectant twinkle of his eyes sparked a Universe of potential in my heart and mind.

I never could have imagined where it would all lead.

By the time I'd made Green Smoothies for both li'l homies and their moms and their friends, there was a line forming, wrapping around the block. My partner in crime, Alan Clarke, the author of the comic book chronicling the Black Panthers, he was kickin' it with me that day. We served at least a few hundred Green Smoothies. It was so much fun!

By the end, the greens I'd brought were demolished. Our offer was simple: anybody could have a smoothie, as long as it was green, that was the only rule.

No greens= no smoothie.

No one really complained.

The energy was amazing. It was fun, people had mad questions, the most poignant being, "Can I make this at home?"

I told them "Yes", and they told me there was nowhere nearby to get the things they needed. I pointed to the food co-op on the corner. "My mama don't shop there, it's too expensive," my little friend told me. The successful co-op, though supporting some aspects of food access in the community, was not a good fit for this family and many others in their situation. I felt defeated, because I'd presented this cool, delicious thing, there was definitely interest, but now no definitive pathway to the prescription. I'd done what so many other folks trying to do good had done, teased at a solution but only provided a cute novelty at a healthy living fair in the hood, an area filled with the traumas created by the racial and economic inequities of systems designed to lock people out of maximizing their energy here on the planet.

One thing I learned during my work at People's Grocery was that wherever people cannot gain easy access to healthy food, their energy and outcomes are being controlled by forces that have plans for them. "You can't get healthy food, you can't organize your mind or your temper or your health? Fine, we have a place for you."

Are there no prisons?
Are there no work camps?
Are there no early graves?

When I left that conversation with the little hearty boy who had the charm, vigor and positive outlook of a resourceful kid from depression-era America—the one who arrives in the narrative with very little, but with hard work and a supportive community ends up successful and whole—when I thought about his diabetes, his mom, the expensive co-op at the corner named after a renowned South African who changed the world, yet the mammas in the community can't afford to walk in and buy a banana, when I thought about all that, Horatio Alger quickly disappeared in a plume of smoke, and the reality of neo-slavery America, where li'l homie resides, where all the families Alan and I made smoothies for that day, reside took its place.

As we stood there and tried to figure out the conundrum, I told him, "We'll figure something out." I said that even though I knew... from long hours sitting at that large wooden table at People's Grocery pouring over books chronicling the history of West Oakland, the Black Panthers, their breakfast program, J. Edgar Hoover's outrageously revealing statement that the Panthers posed the greatest threat to America because they were feeding Black children... even though I'd read that counties across America know how many prison beds to plan for years out by looking at the reading scores of our children in 3rd grade (my little inspiration was about that age)... if he couldn't organize a healthy meal every day, didn't keep his diabetes under control, how would he fare in school...was he a pipeline prison candidate?

It's not depression-era America, no one is coming to help the poor reclaim dreams and humanity. The plan for the poor and Black is prison and slavery.

I couldn't stand the thought of his bright twinkling eyes growing dim because of diabetes and lack of living food and the consequences of all that juxtaposed the other realities of his circumstances.

Diabetes is a highly curable illness. With proper diet and consistent access to the right foods, he could beat it, and so could his mom.

With at least one Green Smoothie a day, that would be just the beginning of a lifetime of proper health management. Food could become his medicine.

Alan and I cleaned up and broke down.

I loaded in, closed the hatch to the car and said "bye" to my new friends. My heart was heavy, and my mind was buzzing. For the first time I realized that if every child in the city had access to at least one nutrient-dense Green Smoothie a day, the chances of focusing and concentrating in school, completing assignments, not cutting up and misbehaving because of hunger, not reaching for Cheetos or other junk food... their chances for a healthy, balanced life would be so much greater. Diabetes and obesity could be a thing of the past. The cute little hearty boy who spent the afternoon zipping up alongside our booth on his bike, and keeping us entertained, promoted our work to the community and became fast friends with us, he would really, really have a chance to make it.

Eldridge Cleaver wrote, "Our children are being organized into their poverty through hunger."

Fifty years later, add a diet of junk food, brain-altering flavor enhancers, sugary drinks and breakfast and lunchroom food that is prepackaged then shipped in from China... today we have a disaster.

Today our children are being organized into the school to prison pipeline, away from freedom, away from options, away from the opportunities that every child in America should have—an opportunity for a life with hope.

When I left and told my little buddy that we'd work it out, I meant it.

I still do.

KETCHUP IS NOT A VEGETABLE

My father was Horatio Alger... or at least the kind of character made famous by the Horatio Alger, the 19th century writer who chronicled through his fiction the archetype of the poor boy who works his way up from very little to achieve great riches, respect and love from the community. When my dad was a kid, America was still a place where this could happen. America was a place where the ethos and consciousness of many of its citizens understood and valued equal participation.

Born in 1946 in Raymar Alabama, my father was the son of bona fide country beauty. Mama Baby, as she was known, was the daughter of African and Blackfoot Native American folk who sharecropped the land at Pine Level, a tiny, rural community a stone's throw from Montgomery. They worked, lived, ate and breathed country life, country air and had simple down-home ways.

After a brief tryst with a handsome, married, middle class businessman from the neighboring town, once she found herself in the family way, Baby was promptly abandoned to deal with the situation on her own.

So though he would carry the Curry name, my father's rearing, his loving, his spiritual development and common sense understanding of the world around him, would come from his mother's people, the Guice clan. When my father was old enough for his mother to realize that he was "different" or "special", as I've heard it called, it was with a broken heart and a head held high with hope that she left him temporarily to go find work in Detroit, Michigan. Her intention was to sow the seeds of a life that held the promise of more opportunity than the meager existence she could eek out of Jim Crow, on the red clay of Alabama. She wanted to organize an environment where a boy like her son, Charles Henry, could be well educated and reap fully the benefits of what seemed to his family and community to be a sharp, gifted mind.

Like many young, single mothers, through her focused determination and hard work, she blazed a pathway for my father's education and a future for him that would exceed anything she could ever dream of for herself.

While she was in Detroit, my father was left in the care of his grandparents, Mama Deah and Daddy Morgan. During the days he ran with his older cousins. One afternoon his destiny unfolded when on a short visit back home, Mama Baby put some money in the hands of my dad's eldest girl cousin. "Ya'll go on down to the store and get some candy n' things. Make sure Charles Henry get some too."

I imagine that my grandmother's strategy was born of the idea that providing candy money for all of the kids, would mean that her own love, her only child at the time, who she missed terribly and was working diligently to be reunited with once things came together in Detroit, well he would definitely get some.

As fate would have it, things didn't quite come together the way Mama Baby had planned. Instead of happily buying the candy and sharing with my father, his cousin bought the candy and passed some around to every one of the kids except my father. When he protested a squabble broke out and little Charles Henry was pushed and rolled down into a ditch.

While the other children continued on down the road back to the farm, eating, drinking and enjoying the fruits of his mother's labor, their voices became distant echoes and my father was left to contemplate his lot.

He shared this story with me and I'll share it with you in his own words.

"Lying in the ditch, crying over the fact that my cousins all had more stuff than I.

We'd just left the store and they had Igey Mikes and drinks and maybe even some candy. I got to drink a sip from them, if one of them felt like sharing. I had to ask them and they had the power to say no and often did. I cried in that ditch and said "one of these day I won't have to ask nobody for nothin'. And then I proceeded to live my life intentionally with a plan to get to that point where I wouldn't ever have to again."

My father was probably fours year old when all of this happened. And with the clarity and zeal we often experience when we are deeply wounded by the ones we love and trust, my father used his wound and his pact of *to never have to ask nobody for nothin'* as rocket fuel to catapult himself from that ditch, to the highest ranking member of any and every school he attended. Charles Henry, who became Chuck or Charles once he moved to Chicago, had so much athletic, social and academic success by the time he graduated from college that he was courted by Oxford University to join the coveted Rhodes Scholarship program and also had invitations from the University of Chicago and Northwestern to complete his graduate education.

He chose Northwestern, where he completed his Masters in accounting and finance. When I asked him why he chose not to follow the path of Rhodes Scholarship (which must have been a thrilling opportunity for this child from the red dust of rural Alabama) he related this.

"Your mother and I had a son and you were on the way. I'd been so impressed with the impact of not having my father in my life or being raised by him, that there was no way I could even consider studying abroad and leaving my little family such a long distance. I wasn't ever going to go live anywhere that I couldn't take you all."

Running into li'l homie on 7th and Peralta made me think a lot about my father, the circumstances of his life, the players and agents that supported his opportunities, as well as my country. The United States of America.

Like many of us who get so caught up in the story of our day to day, I probably never would have thought about many of the facts of my own lineage the choices and decisions of my mother, my father, my grandmother going to Detroit back in the 50's... or the world that supported these choices... the USA attitude back in those days that said "if there was a will there was a way" and that it would be a waste, no matter what color or how impoverished, for a mind like my father's to go to waste...he must have every opportunity to thrive and organize his energy into the great miracle of a healthy successful, positive life...raise a family if he wanted to and participate fully as a healthy, contributing member of society and the world.

That afternoon on 7th and Peralta and meeting that bright, beautiful boy...li'l homie, made me deal with the fact that that time had come and gone. Somewhere, somehow, something had gone terribly, terribly wrong.

My father chose to pursue a career in marketing and advertising. I guess because it was competitive and interesting enough, while still being super stable and potentially lucrative. In the seventies, while we lived in Chicago and he worked at Proctor and Gamble, my father would come home every night and we'd have dinner at a large dining room table my mother'd procured from an antique shop and brought home to accommodate me and my brother's school buddies.

Back in those days, our classmates were from parts of the world where the US government was making mischief, doing the things that tear up communities, families and homes, entire countries, under the name of "freedom and American ideals." Some were from Mexico, Puerto Rico, the Philippines, others from Cambodia, Vietnam, Burma, and other occupied zones.

Like a lot of kids do after school we gathered to do home work. Since our mom was one of the only mom's who didn't work and was cool with them chillin', our place was the spot. Our friends would end up staying for board games and at some point my mom would get a request from one or all of us about them staying for dinner. Mom was ahead of us, she'd already talked to their moms .

The night would culminate with all of us eating together as a family at that table.

Those were great times.

It was at that table, on a street called Belle Plaine, where I heard the stories of an American community, South Chicago, all bundled up in a neat package as seen by my mom and dad—young parents, two kids really, who had been childhood sweethearts—who grew up during a time when folks believed that anybody could achieve anything in this country, as long as they rolled up their, sleeves, worked hard and stayed late. The only way you couldn't make it in America, is if you were lazy. Of course Black folks and people of color had to work harder to make it, but you could still make it.

To me, that was America.

And it seemed, at least to me, from mom and dad's stories, because people had come from so many places to enjoy a better world and here we were, enjoying that better world, it seemed to me, that America was a place that would continue to feel that way. Continue to feel that everyone deserved an opportunity and that everyone in this country felt that way. After all, there was so much movement in the 50s, 60s and 70s. People like my grandmother were migrating every day from one part of the US to the other, knowing that where they were going held one thing they could count on, hope. There was an agreement that America would become more inclusive, more prosperous, more egalitarian—at least it seemed that way.

So there we were at that table, the motley lot of us and we'd all listen as my parents transported us back to their world, Post-World War II, Baby Boom Chicago. It was a living, breathing, mystical moment where for a time, America was beautiful and proud and hopeful and strong. Not because of its army or its stupid meddling wars, but because of the people who agreed that this place would be better. My parents would share the most beautiful, funny and uplifting tales, the way they did with anyone who visited their home, especially at the dinner table, especially about the neighborhood they grew up in.

South Chicago was a small multi-ethnic enclave that ran

along Lake Michigan towards the end of Illinois and bumped up against the Indiana State Line. It was a bustling, thriving and upwardly mobile community that stood in the long shadows of the Chicago Steel Mill.

"You had everybody," my mother would say. "The Greeks, German folks, Mexicans, Chinese, Japanese, Polish, Hungarian, and of course our folks were pouring in everyday because of the lynchings Down South. And there were all kinds of food. On one side mama owned a BBQ restaurant and bar, and on the other you had Frank's tacos. We all lived there together and everybody got along. You had the rail lines, the steel mill, the port. You never had to leave unless you wanted to because anything you needed was right there. It was like we existed in our own world. You were every neighbor's child, you didn't talk back to grown people and you had respect. I mean, we had a neighborhood drunk who would fall down in the street, I mean pass out DRUNK with a capital D and somebody, a neighbor or one of the guys comin' home late from work at the mill, would cover him up so he wouldn't get sick. We weren't even really a part of the rest of Chicago. We were South Chicago. It was beautiful."

One of these nights, long after we'd finished eating, my mother shared with us the story of a sunny afternoon where she and her little girlfriends were playing on her porch. An elder neighbor, who'd been enjoying watching them play with their dolls, jump hopscotch and skip rope, called my mother over and asked her to sit down next to her.

"I have something to tell you."

She told my mother about a man, who came to her city and made sure that everyone of her family was taken away, including her.

"They came and put us on the trains and we walked. They put us in long houses...no heat...it was cold, everyone slept in the same area, there was so little food...so many got sick...so many died. Then she rolled up her sleeve and showed me a tattoo of numbers, permanently inked into her skin. This was a very bad

man and this is what he did to me."

The man's name was Hitler. That was how I learned about the genocide of the Jewish people during World War II. My mother's neighbor had survived the camps and had come to the US to start a new life.

I met my own life lessons at this table as well. I'll never forget prepping the condiments for mom's delicious tacos, with the recipe she got from Frank's Taco Stand. It's a combination of chorizo and ground beef. Nowadays it can also be made with vegetarian ingredients, just as delicious. Anyway, it was my job that night to prep the lettuce, tomato, onions and cheese with my dad. Everything was goin' good until I pulled the lettuce out of the fridge. It was soft. I knew that if the lettuce was soft then I was gonna be dispatched to "run to the store"...CHE...across the street.

CHE was short for CHECKER. Story was the painter had run out of red paint so instead of CHECKER, it was known as CHE, so was the owner.

My mother and her favorite command "Run across the street right quick to CHE," was looming someplace in my not too distant future. I didn't wanna put on my shoes and coat and go to CHE's. So I decided to do it my way. I would wing it. Winging it meant hustling the lettuce to the faucet past my dad so he didn't see it AND rinse it so well that a miracle would occur and I'd bring the lettuce back to life. If I couldn't bring the lettuce back to life with the ice-cold-winter-Chicago-tap-water, I'd have to employ some magical thinking and hope no one noticed the wilted, melting lettuce on the platter of otherwise hearty, robust vegetables and cheeses.

When the resurrection did not occur, undaunted, I put the lettuce on the platter and started sliding the knife through green layers of wilt. My father who'd been watching me organize this nonsense the whole time, unbeknownst to me, finally took pity on me and stopped the show. The kitchen rumbled with the boom of his voice, Moses-like, from the other side of the room "Kelly, what are you doing? That lettuce is gone."

What followed was a verbal chain link of "B...b..b..but I, ..it's just...umm...ya' know..." I was busted and embarrassed. Not only was I caught, but I'd let my dad down and I was probably still gonna have to go to the store. My father took my hands in his and pulled my embarrassed chin up to meet his eyes.

"I want you always to remember that whenever you put food in front of someone to eat, that it must be wholesome, these aren't ornaments, the food we serve is for the nourishment of their Body and Soul.

I can't remember whether I had to bear the elements and march off "right quick" to CHE's, but I never forgot my dad's words. I realize now that Belle Plain Avenue and that fabulously large table of my mother's was where I received 90% of my spiritual development as a kid.

It was around that time that my dad shared with us his first experience making money, picking cotton in the fields of a neighboring farm back in the country, at Pine Level.

"I was the first one on the truck. Wasn't even daylight. Soon as we got to the farm, I was off and running, so excited to make some money, make my contribution. I worked all through the day, never took a break, picked more cotton than any of the boys, or men for that matter and when it came time for work to end, I stood there with all my bushels, I was so proud because I had more than anyone, so naturally I assumed I would get more or at least as much. So I waited as he made his way down the line and I saw him pulling out dollars to pay the other men, everyone got a dollar or two, when it came to be my turn he looked down at me and reached down into his pocket, when he pulled a coin out, I knew it must have been a special coin, but when I saw it... I looked at it twice because I thought that my eyes deceived me.

It was a dime.

I was five and I spent alot of time trying to figure out why, if I'd worked just as hard...harder... why I didn't get paid just as much, I'd done just as much...more."

I'll never forget the look on my father's face which expressed the disharmony of the experience and this new feeling I had in my belly that my father had been hurt as a young boy. That he'd been hurt and exploited. That he'd been betrayed by the adults in his life, all of them—the neighboring farm owner and the other men from his family who didn't stand up for him. It was the first time I felt that way, but it wouldn't be the last. It made me so sad and angry and for the first time I felt true helplessness. Something in me wanted to be the person that went back in time and protected him.

In my world, every adult in my life was looking to protect me, not exploit me or trick me or steal my energy. It was through these stories that I realized how unlike my life was compared to the two people who had brought me into the world and what a complex place America was. There were parts of their stories that I loved. Trust me, I would have traded anything to be a part of that world they lived in as kids. But things like that farm story or like my mom's mother having mistreated her or the other things... It seemed to me as a kid hearing these stories, it was my belief that we were moving towards a world where there would be more protection for children and community.

Not less.

The safety around me said so, the safety of my community said so. And the fact that we were living in my parents vortex of positivity and baby boom abundance said so.

In 1979, everything in my life attested to it.

And I think that somehow, so many years later, when I ran into little homie on the corner of Peralta and 7th, the same corner that Marcus Garvey organized on in the 30's and the Black Panthers organized on in the 60's and 70's, I think all the lessons and the stories that I'd heard at that table, and my own my little buddies... kids whose families were taking refuge here from all over the world whose moms were struggling to make ends meet...like my grandmother had...so my Pop could make something of his life... something about those stories, that training that I received at that table... all the love, our laughter... what I believed America was... and what it certainly was not... made me make a promise to li'l homie that had its roots in justice, common sense and love.

About a year or so after we moved to Belle Plaine, Ronald Reagan was elected to the highest office in the land. He announced on TV one afternoon that ketchup was a vegetable.

So was relish.

So was mustard.

Relish and ketchup and mustard would replace the vegetables that the American government had promised public school breakfast and lunch programs when the Black Panthers shamed them into feeding children school lunches and breakfasts just a few years earlier.

My mother shook her head and sighed, "Lord have mercy. I'll just be damned..."

That was when another America started to take shape for me. One where every night, on television, from the nightly news and Mork and Mindy, people who looked like me, my brother, my friends were profiled as criminals, lazy, lawbreakers and losers.

The steady stream of propaganda coached anyone who would listen on the terrors of "inner cities," "Black Crime," "black-on-black crime" and the evils of somebody called "The Welfare Queen." She lived in Chicago, cheated the system, bought Cadillacs and Mercedes with her welfare checks and had more and more children at the expense of hardworking taxpayers. Anyone with any sense should resent her because she was lazy, liked to lay up and have babies, so she could collect more welfare... so she could drive her Mercedes to the market and buy steak and lobster for her "welfare babies."

This was the nightly news—American media—shaping the opinions and thoughts of one citizen against the other, building fear and sowing the seeds of discord, weaponizing race and class when less than twenty years years prior, Dr. King had shared his dream of folks coming closer together.

The federally funded "bootstrap" programs in our Chicago neighborhoods that had sent folks back to school and gave people a second chance at participating if they were high school dropouts or had had struggles with drugs or otherwise peripheralizing circumstances were cut and replaced with, get this, nothing.

People were left out in the cold and the energy in the country not-so-slowly started to change. Reagan would come on TV and say things like, "We are going to take things back to the good old days," and my mother would get that same tone in her voice that she had when the ketchup as a vegetable thing happened and she'd look at me and say, "You know what he's talkin' bout baby don't you? The good ol' days?"

When I didn't answer, she'd school me. "He's talkin' about Jim Crow. He's talking about slavery. Lord have mercy." This seemed outlandish to me, but he had said that ketchup was a vegetable and I knew that was nonsense. So maybe mom had a point...but slavery? Jim Crow? How could they do that? Jim Crow was when my father, a child laborer had received a dime for before sun-up to sun-down labor. I couldn't picture me or my brother doing that, or my mom and dad or Michael Jackson or James Earl Jones on an auction block.

Could my mother be right, could they put us back in chains and find a way to pay us nothing for our work?

Could you even make kids work?

Not in America...

The beat continued and the nightly news was doing plenty of reporting about how aimless and lazy Black Americans were and if we could just stop being so paranoid in thinking that there were "conspiracies" working against us that we would truly be able to join the American middle class and things would get better for us.

The mood at our dinner table started to change too. I started hearing words like "propaganda" and we would discuss, especially my parents and their friends, "look how ignorant they make us look on TV these days," and "Why do they always choose the most ignorant Black person in the crowd to comment whenever something happens?"

After Reagan had taken office there were alot of changes in the community too. A depression of spirit hit.

Very quickly, communities and cities in our country that had been organizing and fighting for equity and human rights were flooded with crack cocaine and a gap, a large void began to take shape that created gulfs as big as the Great Lakes that would further disconnect Black folks from white, middle class from poor, and everyone else from everyone else.

That other America, the one where you could roll up your sleeves and work hard and make something of your life, even if you were poor, the one where folks could safely care about one another was receding and the one where folks were being seduced by one of the richest opiate—fear—loomed.

And the poor, they were pariahs, to be discarded, couldn't be trusted.

They were poor because they were wastes of time and energy and belonged at the bottom.

The poor were poor because they were lazy losers and deserved to be poor.

The America of my parents dreams, the beautiful, idyllic stories of their Baby Boom community seemed further and further behind us, as distant and unrealistic as the promise of a job with a great future with US Steel, which slowly downsized until it announced its closing in 1992.

I didn't know it back in those days, as a kid sitting at that table, but all of these things were forming and coloring and shaping and shading the outlines of the world and circumstances of a little boy who would appear on my horizon... and that I would meet thirty plus years later on a street corner in West Oakland.

Somehow,I would enter, the intolerably bleak void that he stood in, called out from and dwelled within and meeting him would change the world for me. It would be that gleam in his eyes, the sound of his voice, his laughter and the fact that my heritage and teachings and ancestral traditions told me that even though we'd only met once, that he was my brother, my cousin, my nephew... my son....

I'd see all too clearly how Reagan's promise and my mother's fears had come true. He said "We are going to take things back to where they used to be." They made good on that one..

That boy, that child, was mine... he belonged to me and every other American that had been convinced of his worthlessness. The programming and propaganda of the nightly news and America's original, shameful wounds of land theft and enslavement of the African had slowly and methodically coerced Americans into a solid hatred and fear of poverty and Blackness.

Once and for all... obliterating any sense that this place would be different... that this place would be better.

As my father shared with us at our dinner table, from his training at Kellogg School of Management, Northwestern University, "All you have to do to make something the truth is repeat it over and over and over and over again. One day, people wake up believing it is true and that it has always been true.."

Programming.

That's what commercials are. That's what advertising does. Program us.

Smoking is sexy.
Indians are red.
Drink Cow's Milk for Calcium
Coca Cola is good for you.
Trust a man in a white coat.
Beware the Welfare Queen.
Beware Black youth.

By the time I run into li'l homie on 7th and Peralta, Reagan's peeps are reaping the dividends on their promise to "take things back to the good old days." and I see what I could not have imagined when I was eleven and my mother pronounced the outcomes... Jim Crow... Slavery.

Neo-slavery would not be a public auction block in the public square. It would happen behind God's back and manifest through an elaborately tight weave of manufactured consent on behalf of Americans who forgot all about Martin Luther King's vision of equal economic participation for all races. His poor people's campaign had been flipped to the war on the poor launched by Reagan and his boys.

The tools:
1. A completely chemicalized, weaponized food system that makes people sick, disorients them and dumbs them down.
2. School systems that organize youth into despair, despiritualization, and hopelessness.
3. Corporate sponsored, locally run correctional facilities and police forces who act as herders for youth into local justice systems as first step to a life of free labor behind the bars of state and federal prisons. Neo slavery.
4. An American populous that through corporate control, media, advertising, and materialism is being herded and does not have time or resources to unravel the truths of the manipulation and the reasons for it all: control of energy and resources in order for a few folks to control most of the wealth and resources in the land.

In 1974 Gil Scott Heron released his prophetic Winter In America.

It took us a while. But Gil knew that we'd make it. Now here we are. 44 years later, we are living it. Our children stand within the void and Horatio Alger is long gone.

FEED THE 5,000

After meeting the boy on the corner of 7th and Peralta at The Bikes For Life in West Oakland, I made the case for People's Grocery to really invest in supporting the healing of community through Green Smoothies. When I got the green light to purchase our own Vitamix, we continued to utilize the map presented by the elder in her directive that we "move nutrition through the community." The original Green Smoothie brigade was my artist friend Alan, Chris Crosby (People's Grocery fellow), Patrick Cody-Carrese, an intern who'd come to work with us that summer, and Paula Beal.

I'd first seen Paula's bright, full, smiling face on the cover of HOPE Collaborative's community outreach piece and when we met I felt I'd known her forever. I said a few words about the project and she was in love. Because of Paula's connections in the world of human rights in Oakland at large, she was able to make a case for HOPE Collaborative to take on smoothies as part of their Corner Store Conversion Project. Paula's complete agreement, as a mother, grandmother and community ally, that Green Smoothies were a perfect addition to shops and stores in our communities because of the lack of whole nutrition otherwise available, made me feel like I was on the right track. Her genuine support of our efforts and my burning passion made a big difference in the continuity and validity of the work.

Word spread about the project and that summer we took advantage of every opportunity and every invitation to get those Green Smoothies out into the world, wherever we could: basketball courts, skate parks, public rallies, backyard BBQ's, family festivals. In addition I was also campaigning for the "One Smoothie a Day" for Oakland kids.

I talked smoothie so much that people were sick of hearing about it.

One day my boss called me into her office and in the nicest way possible suggested I ease up a little. I got offended. It sounded to me like I was being accused of being a crazy person.

"I can't stop talking about it until it happens, I don't care who thinks I'm crazy. We can do this. It can work." Years later I realize, humbly, that perhaps she was only trying to protect me and save me from upsetting my colleagues with my obsession. But it was too late, I'd gone to the other side.

I was indeed obsessed with what seemed like such a doable, easy answer.

After all, I was seeing too much suffering. It was needless, hunger-related suffering during my work in West Oakland. And my research was saying that people were hungry for real minerals, nutrients and dense proteins. All the things you had when you put greens, fruit 'n water in a Vitamix and hit 'blend'. Not to mention that a lot of these things were being thrown out in the back of supermarket dumpsters because they were one or two days beyond expiration or simply "didn't look good enough" to sell.

I could afford to look crazy, what I could not afford, what my heart couldn't stand, was the idea of not seeing this project through, the idea walking away without having fulfilled the doable thing of making sure kids had access to at least one Green Smoothie a day didn't feel right. I'd made a promise that sunny day in West Oakland, and even though I might never see that kid again, I had to do my best to fulfill it.

We had to do our best to work it out.

At the end of that summer, People's Grocery, in partnership with Green Peace, pulled off the very first International Green Smoothie Day at the Green Peace warehouse in West Oakland. Special thanks to my friend Georgia Hirsty for supporting that idea through to its manifestation.

At this moment, two things happened.

1. My friend and street smoothie ally, Ms. Paula Beal, suggested we call the campaign of healing community through Green Smoothies How Are You Healing Today?

2. I got a call from someone at the city asking if we'd like to participate in an international festival to end food waste.

All we had to do was what we'd been doing... make Green Smoothies... for 5,000 people.

"You think you guys can pull it off?"

Cut to downtown offices of StopWaste, a reliable local funder of a lot of the Food Justice work that goes on in Oakland.

It was a planning meeting for Feed The 5,000.

Feed The 5,000 represented an opportunity to make meals for folks, using food that would otherwise end up in the dumpster, because it was unattractive and therefore unsalable.

In America every year, billions of pounds of edible food end up as waste, even though a quarter of households do not have enough food to make it through to the end of the month.

This was THE opportunity to show how a few freshly-harvested greens from our city gardens, "ugly fruit" and teamwork could make magic in health and prosperity through the Green Smoothie. So of course I jumped in and pledged the support of the organization. We assembled volunteers and organized fruit and greens from our own garden at People's Grocery, Cal Hotel and other sources. On the day of October 15, 2014, we blended over 5,000 smoothies downtown Oakland at Frank Ogawa Plaza for the people of Oakland.

The headline of OaklandNorth.net read "Feed The 5000 Serves Free Smoothies And Soup, Satisfies Thousands."

The article continued: "This was the first Feed The 5,000 event in the United States, which took place at Frank Ogawa Plaza in Oakland on Saturday. More than 5,000 servings of lunch were prepared out of fruits and vegetables that would otherwise have been wasted."

That afternoon, as I watched an army of volunteers peel bananas, chop and blend greens and hand out ice-cold Green Smoothies into the hands of people lined up hundreds deep, I thought of my little twinkly-eyed homie from West Oakland,

and hoped that this next step would get me closer to realizing my doable goal. If we could pull this together, why couldn't we pull it together in local schools, so children could have one Green Smoothie a day?

I was somewhere closer to that place on the map where this would be a reality... my guides and inspirations were his bright eyes and my community elder who told me "THIS is what you need to be doing."

When I left People's Grocery six months later, I took my green-smoothies-as-a-human-right dream and How Are You Healing Today? with me and I joined forces with Planting Justice.

My time at People's Grocery, rich and full with many lessons and an understanding of a West Oakland being punished for yielding the cradle of a Revolution for Black People and other People of Color internationally in the 60's, was an integral part of my decolonization and I will be forever thankful.

I left however, with a focused mission, to move as much nutrition through the community as possible, culminating with children having access to at least one Green Smoothie a day... citywide.

THAT WHICH IS FREE AND ABUNDANT

But through what mechanism, path or magic could I possibly bring Green Smoothies to 50,000 children of Oakland? In one sense such a goal is hardly out of our reach. The math is simple 10 x 5000. We fed 5000 in one day. What would it take us to do ten times that, every day? To do that we will need to harness the abundant energy that is all around us.... in the children, the parents, the teachers... in the schools, the stores the streets... in the greens, the fruits, the herbs.... in the land, the water, the air.

I began to think deeply about the complex and wondrous energy all around us and my mother and father teaching me that the purest, most abundant energy in the world is the power of love... a gift from God.

That teaching reminded me of Nikola Tesla.

I became enchanted with Tesla about 11 years ago. A great friend of the family, a Hungarian engineer/ boat builder/ mechanic/ you-name-it-he-can-do-it, he introduced me to Tesla.

He was stunned when I told him I'd never heard of him. "Ahh yes," he said. "America, what they teaching the kids about electricity?! Ahhh I forget, America pretending that Edison is responsible for connecting to the electricity."

From our friend I learned that JP Morgan and Thomas Edison had essentially hired Tesla to organize the innovation of electricity through the alternating current, technology which Tesla channeled through his remarkable abilities as a mystical scientist. It was important to Tesla that the information and technology be free and abundant.

What Tesla did not—what he could not have known—was that the organizers he'd teamed up with wanted to collect on his inventions... forever. And cut him out of the deal completely.

They were successful.

Subsequently, even though the blueprint for the world we

are living in today was created by Nikola Tesla...most people do not know that he ever existed

Tesla's ministry was organizing and liberating connections and channels to energy, free of charge, so that humanity could know peace and prosperity and ascend to spiritual heights here on earth

I know that it is God's wish for us to enjoy the beautiful bounty of this beautiful magical Earth, in all of her glory and diversity. This includes access to foods that keep us healthy, strong and fully functioning.

This organic health, balance and inspiration yield access to more ease, more beauty, more abundance and a beautiful world, far beyond the realms of our wildest dreams.

Unfortunately the systems that govern our society are tied up in harnessing and selling what is organic, free, pure and God given: energy.

Not just electricity, but all energy, including human energy.

It is why the African, "freed" from slavery in America around 1864, is enslaved en masse in prisons across North America.

It is why our little African-American boy living in West Oakland, chugging down smoothies and cautious about his diabetes, cherubic and full of life, vigor, melanin and strength, is being groomed for a life of enslavement. The grooming tools are poverty, miseducation and a lack of the living nutrition that would fully excite his brain, mind, spirit and imagination to its full potential and organize a host of other opportunities, simply because his brain, body, mind and spirit are fully alive and excited, curious and engaged in living.

Under the current system, one of the only apparent pathways illuminated are leading him directly to a life of enslavement via the Prison Industrial Complex, which, like JP Morgan and Edison's electrical grids and power lines, will harness his energy and sell the products of his labor for the rest of his days.

Under the systems that govern this society, human energy,

must be harnessed, controlled and sold to the highest bidder. The other items on this laundry list of natural, dynamic forces to exploit for capital gain include wind energy, solar energy, energy from rivers and the oceans and mighty Great Lakes of the Midwest, the energy of plants, the energy of the Earth and the energy of anyone getting up every day to go to a job they cannot stand, so they may put food on the table and participate in other ways of holding these unsustainable systems together.

For me, getting to know more about Tesla—his mystically guided path—meant understanding his heart and his dreams, and how terribly he was treated because he worked to share insights and knowledge that he knew would liberate humankind from the endless sufferings of slavery. At the same time, living in and near gardens and hearing, as well as seeing the natural, abundant, healing systems of the Earth, converted me from someone frustrated and confused and hurt by the limits and boundaries of our communities and opportunities, to an evangelist for the liberation of energy and light found in even a single blade of grass.

The miracle of energy cannot be harnessed and sold unless we agree to let it be. Currently, because we are participating with these systems, steeped in the belief that they are the only way, we appear to be in agreement with them... including the systems that keep our young, innocent—but ill—protagonist, (li'l homie) locked in a pipeline with outcomes such as demise of his health and lack of opportunities.

Healing our bodies, returning to natural patterns of sleeping and eating and being in community and engagement with the Earth... whatever that looks like for you, may be the first steps towards sustainability and balance.

For me, it started with tapping into my own abundant energy field by harvesting greens with my own hands, from local soil and herbs and local seasonal fruit and blending it all into a power pack of life and richness.

The more I participate in these healing exercises, the more I understand that the Earth is beckoning us to heal our ways, our practices, what we put in our bodies... with her. One cannot truly happen without the other.

Not participating in holding these systems together will not be an option for most people.

That is reasonable.

But for those who have had enough, for those who are interested in organizing something else... something living, that feels good and whole, the first step could be to learn to conjure and command your own energy.

To engage in the shift that will support the lives of young people like the boy I met on the street corner years ago, we must first heal our own bodies and reconnect to natural systems. Healing our bodies, returning to natural patterns of sleeping and eating and being in community and engagement with the earth... whatever that looks like for you, may be the first steps towards sustainability and balance.

Every response will not be as radical as mine. I mean, I don't expect folks to go out and bust systems, stand on street corners and sell and give away electricity in a cup, but with one Green Smoothie a day, undernourished children and many adults are tapping into the wellspring of their own energy, less disease and a greater likelihood of succeeding—away from the prisons and work camps where there are beds and lives of hopelessness and despair waiting.

PLANTING JUSTICE

When Haleh Zandi, co-founder of Planting Justice and Director of Education, hired me, she later said it was because of my passion.

She wanted to support my activism.

She and the organization did... still do.

It was through nurturing these kinds of relationships, with people whose hearts are genuinely with moving progress along for the sake of the folks who have been forgotten and marginalized, that I realized that on our own, we're pretty limited, but with homies in the struggle, united, working interdependently towards the same goals, we can truly be a force that can change the world.

Working with Planting Justice catapulted me into a wild, motley crew of activists... young, old, white, Afro-Native, Indigenous, and everything in between... who were doing just this. And together, we got a lot done. We built gardens, organized educational forums in-house and for community at large, fed high school students weekly, plotted love through food and connection to the earth and her medicines and made sure there were places for men who had been thrown away by society to make a decent living and always have the support of a community that truly believed in them and reaffirmed that there was nothing they could not achieve.

Many had served hard time in places like San Quentin. The experience of working side by side with folks from such different walks of life, but supporting the same missions on the front lines, gave me a lot of unanticipated lessons and the kind of growth as an activist and helped me see things about Kelly that I truly needed to know and understand about Kelly.

Going into San Quentin, as a volunteer with Planting Justice, changed my world. Sitting in workshops with brothers who are doing hard time for offenses from their youth, and have them connect the dots on their lack of sound nutrition as young men... as children, and realize that they were set up by the Hoovers of our country, to be deprived and housed in jails... it changed my heart and created even more of a sense of purpose and mission.

It was Hoover who told America that she could not "stand the rise of a Black Messiah." To this end, food deserts and starvation are handy tools.

There was no way, after spending time in the vegetable garden at San Quentin, built by Planting Justice and men imprisoned by the State of California, that I could ever doubt the role that food insecurity plays in destabilizing and blocking human creativity and energy.

The afternoons at the prison gave my work back in Oakland, at high schools and Juvenile Justice camps, with young people who still had a chance not to end up in the pipeline, another added dimension of immediacy. Training high school students to build gardens; supporting an understanding that an everyday touching of the earth could build health and healing; the importance of bees to our environment and how to harvest honey; the beauty of harvesting fruits and greens that they grew and making smoothies for the student body and organizing themselves to work in cooperation with nature and their community-all these things took on a whole new level of emergency to me. Ironically, I thought back to my original Earth work, in Harlem, New York City... and reminded myself of so many of the lessons I'd learned back then. "Do your best and don't blame yourself when you've done the best you can."

But still, there is that creeping reality that your best isn't always good enough, and the first time one of those things you hope will never happen... happens. It was my turn to live this lesson and put this advice to the test. I walked into juvie and saw one of our students on lockdown.

I can't describe the feeling.

"Don't I know you from the Smoothie booth at McClymonds?" He asked with a beautiful smile on his face, bright, gorgeous, brown skinned child, pointing at me like we'd both just won the lottery. Then I guess as he realized where he was and why we were there... the shame set in... I gave him a fist bump, since there's no hugging allowed, smiled at him with all the love I had and told him I was happy to see him, regardless of where... and that I hoped he took the time to enjoy the garden the other boys had built with Planting Justice. I asked him to make sure to come to class next time so we could make smoothies together.

Seeing him there made me feel like the system was working faster than we ever could and I didn't wanna seem sad, but I was so disappointed in the world that had failed this boy, a world I am a part of, a world I participate in.

I felt like I'd walked into one of my nightmares. It's the last thing you want for any kid, to go down that road, but especially one whose life you had hoped to touch.

All those years ago when I was working with Derek Jeter's organization at Jackie Robinson After-school Program in Harlem, Derek's father, a wise, beautiful Black brother, told me something I often have to remind myself of while doing this work.

He said "You do the best you can. Always. And accept that you can't do everything. You're not gonna reach every kid, but you never stop doing your best, to try." On days when you walk into a juvenile prison and see a kid that you worked with on the outside... those are the days you need that kind of wisdom and support. Otherwise you can start to go a little crazy... in a bad way... and hopelessness can start to set into your work.

These things can cloud that wellspring of passion that used to seem endless.

PAULA

Even though we'd segued to doing Smoothies once a week at McClymonds High School, a project that continues to this day under the leadership of my old friend and colleague Anthony Forrest, someone who served 25 years and came out to turn his life into pure magic, and I even entered into talks to support creation of a cafe at the school, with a full Smoothie Bar, a project I am still working on with OUSD and the amazing Librarian at that school, Leah Jensen, things were very bleak on the home front.

Right now housing, like food, is extremely insecure for many families here in the Bay Area. This is because of gentrification.

It hit home when my dear friend Paula Beal was evicted from her home.

An African American elder, with no place to go, she took to living in the backseat of her children's truck. I couldn't believe that it was happening. I knew in my heart though, that I would be next.

The greed afoot in the Bay Area has created a climate of inhumanity that I have only read about in history texts, and classic literature. I have never lived through it, or seen it happen quite like this.

So on an evening in April of 2016, I met Paula at the Taco Bell by my house, and gave her and her family $70 for a hotel for the night.

It was just one night... but what about the next night and the next? Paula was trying to be strong for me, I could see it, but the image of seeing her in that backseat, with her grandchildren no less... houseless on a cold, rainy night with nowhere to go...

I went home, got under the covers and cried.

My tears may have been a healing release of the intense frustration and anger I was feeling, seeing my beautiful, passionate friend who'd supported work for healing... in the backseat of a truck, with her grandchildren who were also without a home... my tears however, were not gonna help find Ms. Paula a place to rest her head.

I had to do whatever I could to support a better situation.

So after a few days of helping out in small ways, I sat down and wrote a letter to friends.

Here it is.

***

Fighting with Love... For Paula Beal
by Kelly Curry

It's Thursday, April 13, 2016.

Last night, Susie Chang opened the door to her home around 9:45, as Catherine and I walked Paula and her belongings, a little carry on stuffed with clothes and a cloth sack filled with her paperwork, indoors.

Paula Beal is smallish framed, usually energetic and bold in presence. This night though, she is tired. I'm seeing that in between the stress of her current situation and her failing health, exacerbated by her current situation, she's lost weight. There is a thinness to her usually full, robust cheeks that makes my heart sink and it scares me. Despite it all, she is apparently thankful and relieved as she breathes a sigh of relief, giving a slight smile as she comes out from the cold into the warmth of Susie's home.

Paula is elder-sister-mom to so many of us who engage in a human movement for freedom and equity in the Bay Area... one that has as many dimensions as the Power we fight has hounds with mighty jaws and razor-sharp teeth.

The teeth either kill you or make you stronger.

One thing is for sure, once you feel the snap of the jaws coming down, it doesn't matter whether you survive, you will not emerge the same as when you got involved... and at some point, you will wish you hadn't.

As we walk into Susie's home, someone who only

yesterday was a stranger, and whose only real connection to me is that she too loves Paula, and we negotiate awkwardly where to arrange Paula's things, it dawns on me that the only energy powerful enough to bend, maim, and soften the bite of these enormously sharp and jagged killing machine-teeth, with mighty jaws that work to devour us all... is love.

Something that if we seed, sow and harvest in abundance... can save us and rock this earth's foundation.

Love is the beautiful, moving, fluid, balmy energy that is giving us the courage to move out of our normal routine and edge ourselves out into places that we do not know this evening, with strangers who meet at the intersection of fear and anger and hurt and "but if I don't do this then what will happen to Paula tonight... and if not me then who?"

"If we do nothing... who is next?"

This night, love has us taking risks and facing the fear that the thing that is happening to our brothers and sisters and neighbors... elders in community, like Paula, who check for us when we are down, have the wisdom to pick us up with a smile or a pep talk or just a sweet, big hug when we are feeling low or weak... if this thing can happen to them, then it can happen to anyone.

Including us.

Me.

You.

This night, one of us is caught up in the snap and grind of those mighty jaws... snarling behind the white teeth. And she is the most vulnerable of us all.

This night we are united to keep Paula loved and healed and nourished and safe in the midst of the Bay Area housing crisis that is despiritualizing our city, devouring historic residents, chewing folks up and spitting us out to land where we land... no matter whether there is breath in our bodies... no matter whether our Souls sit silently watching while our families, friends and loved ones light candles and sing songs, send silent prayers in vigils that mark the spaces where the machinations of greed snatched up our human bodies and new people walk the paths that we paved by walking... smiling in the sunshine that at one time shined down on us.

Right now, my friend, mentor and partner in community healing is homeless.

She carts her few belongings out of her kids's truck, when we scoop her to take her to Susie's this night... the one they share with their grandchildren, they are also homeless... looking battle-worn but hopeful and happy for some refuge, no matter how temporary, Paula climbs into my car and we begin to strategize. Next steps... Raise funds? Seek temporary housing? In this moment permanency seems a strange, expensive, elusive dream. The whole time I'm thinking "what about tomorrow night?" And for the first time in my life, I'm really scared.

I am wondering now, like I often do, how things got to be this way. Hardworking people, elders and their children's children, vital players in our communities who campaign together and build new worlds together, are having to make it the best way they can, in the streets, living in cars and vans and trucks, relying on public spaces and restaurants and the kindness of strangers, to use their toilets and restrooms, bathing in sinks. These are people I love... know... work with... laugh with... plot Green Smoothie bombings on street corners for babies in West Oakland who reside in food deserts throwing seed bombs and the kids smile at her and don't curse at all when they see she's on their block because they love and respect her... while many of the pieces of this world seem to crumble around us... Paula remains vigilant and solid.

Her love-justice work sits at the intersection of the moment that makes and breaks us all: food and housing.

Now ironically, in spite of the sleepless nights of planning and coalition-building to ensure the health and well-being of young people and families throughout Oakland via the Healthy Corner Store Project with HOPE Collaborative and countless hours volunteering with Just Cause, and People's Grocery back in the day, she is herself without a reliable food system or shelter.

Even though she climbed the stairs to City Hall only days after emerging from the hospital with Just Cause to demand a moratorium on evictions and rent hike (the one Oakland's City Council passed unanimously last week), here I am, calling around to friends and people I barely know asking for a couch... a shared room... when I want a castle with Nebuchadnezzar's gardens to house and nourish my friend and her immaculate soul for healing.

Paula is the one who seeks us out when we disappear from the grinding down that happens in the jaws... when we can't take anymore. She finds us and says, "Baby just rest and love yourself and heal and we'll be here for you."

Despite all of this, right now Paula is in the jaws.

We may not know it, but we are all in the jaws and the teeth are coming for us... all... and if we don't do something they will snap down on us... that something is activating the most powerful force in the world...love for one another... for Paula... right now.

Fight with love for Paula... now.

***

In the moment of writing and distributing this letter to colleagues, friends, strangers, anyone who would listen, I'd done all I could. As fate and destiny would have it, Nicole, a friend and colleague from Planting Justice, read the letter and took Paula in.

They got on marvelously. I was able to turn my attentions to my own troubles.

As far as my situation was concerned, my own housing issues pushed me into purchasing a retrofitted school bus.

In mid-August I moved into it.

I loved it.

Then summer turned to fall and quickly to winter and it got mad cold outside... freezing on the bus. It was during these times that I began to truly think back to my lessons and teachings of America, the ones at the dinner table as a child. And one night on the bus, I distinctly felt my mother, now part of the spirit world tell me "this is what we protected you from...this is what you have never experienced, now you will see and feel and understand."

Still she was with me.

From her dimension, she and my father, protecting me, my family, my partner and our animals, doggies, Play and Sausage.

I am an adventurer, so living on a bus was simply brilliant, but there were times when it was scary... lonely... and even though the experience revolutionized my consciousness around the variety of ways to live, there were those who judged me and wanted to stigmatize me and called me "homeless."

Folks made all kinds of comments, to my face that betrayed a deep sense of hatred and disdain for my situation... for what they took to be poverty juxtaposed my Blackness.

Even though I chose a very dynamic response to a phenomena that is wreaking havoc on the social and cultural, spiritual infrastructure of the Bay Area, when I moved onto the bus, to some people, whose view supports this kind of thinking, I was just another homeless Black woman. In my world view, I was having an artistic, creative adventure, one that I was happy and excited to undertake. It was peppered with inconvenience... but compared to life in other places, life on a cute, funky, retrofitted school bus, in an eclectic urban area with options—let's just say things could have been worse. Even though I never responded to these comments, attitudes and judgments, none of it was lost on me.

My heart and mind considered and mourned the America of my parents childhoods, good ol' South Chicago, where people looked after one another and helped one another. Plus, what if I were a kid, living on a bus with my family, being traumatized and bullied by classmates because I was living differently? I started to look at people living in tents, in cars, in boxes.. buses and open-airing-it in push carts in a completely different way... with more love and understanding, and I began to speak up for them when other people used objectifying, alienating phrases like "homeless," or "street person," or "derelict." I became sensitive to a world I'd generally paid very little attention to, save considering how to support in small ways. Now I knew what I had to do and I heard God's mandate; show love, send love, pray love and be love.

During quiet times on the bus I also considered those late night chats at the table with my family, our friends, and the messages about Black folks and poor people during the early 80s... the bombing of our psyches with the "Welfare Queen" and the beginnings of relentless poverty and the acceptance of "poor" Blacks and poor White trashy Whites and "dirty Mexicans" as the norm in a place that used to support everyone's upward mobility as long as they worked hard... stayed late and weren't lazy.

I started to look around and realize that the people passing the tents by, (that had popped up by the thousands in the Bay Area) that the people with traditional housing have developed a force field which makes them think and believe that somehow they can look down on these folks, when the real fear could be that over night they can BECOME these folks... otherwise why would people let other people live like this... and the children... all of the children climbing out of tents.

It was during this time that I became acutely aware that simple, readily-available access to whole nutrition was a big issue for this community as well, the discarded, overlooked, stepped over and forgotten members of our human community living on the fringes of our society. A huge issue. It may sound nuts, but when you're trying to hold your world together, the most important thing to your body is sound, nutrient dense nutrition that will fulfill your body's needs to support your nervous system, your brain, your heart...steady digestion and most of all a wellspring of hope, since everyone else may have given up on you... including you.

There were many nights, looking for a safe place to dock my bus, that I saw children standing under the freeway, panhandling with their parents for money to buy food. I even ran into a boy one afternoon downtown, "excuse me Miss, do you have a dollar or any change, I'm trying to get money for me and my brothers and sisters so we can eat tonight." I realized that I'd never run into children... not here in the US, begging for money for food, until I came to Oakland... the edge of the world. That all of the children were Black, polite, and had the same story affirmed my understanding that something is wrong. Terribly wrong. When I ran these stories by colleagues, other activists, they usually told me not to worry, because the children were probably trying to get money for drugs or something else besides food. These opinions supported my sense that most middle class folks have little understanding of how many families are food insecure in our city and provided more evidence that demonizing the poor is now the norm.

It also provided kindling for the fire that raged in me regarding providing Green Smoothie kiosks in schools and other places where children hang out on the daily.

In the midst of being witness to these situations, things got real and seriously stressful when Paula, my partner in street magic, was diagnosed with terminal cancer.

Things were so hectic with work... gardening, smoothies, San Quentin, Juvenile Justice, Food Justice workshops AND living on the bus... that all I could do was get updates from Nicole about how Paula was doing... back-and-forth to the hospital feeling better... then getting sick again... using her body, voice and strength to organize power for the people I later realized she knew she was leaving behind...

Finally in late winter, the woman who coined the phrase How Are You Healing Today? was admitted to hospice. Nicole, who had supported Paula through doctors visits, emergency trips to the ER, worked tirelessly to get her placed in a space that gave Paula the support she needed in her vulnerable circumstance, and was the driving force in maintaining a dignified transition for Paula and had become her friend, called me and told me it was time.

I'll never forget the night I drove my bus over to Alameda to see her.

It was so cold outside.

I walked into the room and I could hear her crying out in pain. I held her hand and knew as someone who loved her, that there was nothing I could do, except be there with her. Other folks in the community were there as well. People she'd organized with, Food Justice activists who she worked along side for years. That night, Ashel from SOS Juice, who is now part of Hip Hop Is Green was there, at her side comforting her, stroking her hair, praying with her.

Something happened to me as I watched her and reflected on her last six months. I realized that if we didn't help one another to change the way that things were in this world, then there would be no hope for change.

We were the hope.

We are the hope.

Paula deserved to be in her own home. If it weren't for Nicole she would have left her body while residing at a shelter, a scenario that was suggested by a cold, detached ER doctor during one of their many nights in the hospital emergency room, "take her to a homeless shelter."

She deserved more and again it seemed like the darkness was working faster then we could.

To think just six months ago Paula was a robust, fighting, beautiful woman... working with us on street corners blending smoothies, talking to community, traveling to Washington DC, and working to ensure fair housing rights for all people... now her spirit was leaving her body... leaving us... and I know that the stress of being without a home rushed her to an early end.

As I walked out and faced another cold night on the bus, I warmed myself with the promise that I would use my life's energy to honor the question... How Are You Healing Today? and make sure that Paula's example and legacy lived on.

I drove and parked the bus on Apgar, where my friend Nicole... another Nicole... lived. She told me to crash for the night if I wanted. I had the key, let myself in and went into her little room, full of inspiring books and art chronicling love and struggles internationally for freedom. I peeled off my clothes and charged my phone and got into the bed and wondered what in the world was happening. My understanding those few years earlier that nutrition was lynchpin to sound opportunity to make it in the world was one thing, now I was experiencing the repercussions of what could happen when housing also became an issue. My thoughts were of the children I saw begging for food, children I'd seen climbing out of tents who lived under the freeways and in many tent-cities that were popping up around Oakland, as folks like Paula and me, were displaced because of the greed afoot.

I fell asleep praying for something better for everyone.

I'd traveled a long way from the warm, secure, loving environment where this journey started, Belle Plaine and those beautiful, comforting family dinners. When I thought back to that world, the hope and the sense that America was safe, that we were all safe as long as we were honest and hardworking...the moments before Reagan when our President was the peanut farmer...that was my programming, peace and reasoning... I guess we'd all come a long way. The other end of the dark tunnel created by Reagan and years and years and years of relentless, covert attacks against education, living wages, access to natural foods and a complete co-option of our human systems by corporations...what a nightmare.

What I was seeing, experiencing...living through...would I ever be able to express or describe in a way that was understandable?

Oakland wasn't happening in a vacuum, something inside me said that soon, all of America would be digesting the same poison of gentrification, elder abuse and human rights abuses against children...it only made sense. Everyday I watched people drive by, walk over and pass thousands of homeless people in the streets and do nothing. To them, somewhere, somehow it was justified.

I guess according to the people who didn't know her, Paula, because she relied on public assistance to feed her children when she couldn't make ends meet, was the Welfare Queen they'd warned us about.

Lazy. Losers. Poor because she didn't work and was ignorant.

None of it was real.

None of it had ever been true.

It was all lies and propaganda. Ketchup wasn't a vegetable. Neither was relish or mustard.

Like Edison made us pay for the power that Tesla brought to us in the coils, and pretended he created it... now we got to see where the lies took us and what believing them would do to us.

I closed my eyes before I went crazy and fell asleep praying for something better for everyone.

I awoke to my phone ringing...shocked out of a deep sleep, I recognized Paula's son's voice on the other end. It was 7:00 AM and he was calling to let me know that my friend, Aquarian guide and Smoothie road dog had passed away.

Once again I didn't know how to feel. I went through the motions of calling friends, associates, sent out an email devoid of my usual buoyancy... I was dying inside... becoming numb.

I had my work to hold onto and my goal of moving nutrition through the community and one day seeing smoothies everywhere as a form of sustainable easy nutrition for children and elders. But honestly during the cold of that winter and the death of Paula, preceded by the transition of mother Georgia, another fierce, common sense precious activist spirit, I felt like I was losing ground.

The horizon I'd seen so clearly, where the electrified Green Smoothies were flowing and happy, healthy children and community participated in the diligent, urgent work of healing... seemed more and more obscured by dense fog and storming dark clouds.

These things juxtaposed the fact that I was beginning to understand myself as something of an outlier in the world of Bay Area activism, where call out culture, Facebook manifestoes and grandstanding seemed to be the "true work" of the activist. These things made me regret every sunrise... a feeling I had never known or encountered. I mean, with all the people Ms. Paula had supported and helped, Nicole, a stranger, who had never met her, but felt it was awful that an elder be houseless, was the one who took her in.

I had some serious questions, hurts and agonies around all of these things and they just seemed to be stacking up.

I just didn't know what to do.

For the first time I started thinking about leaving Oakland. For the first time I thought that maybe it was just too much for me. My work, so essential and grounding, had become too dark. I was a long way from the early victories of those West Oakland street corners, the buoyant laughter of the original smoothie crew, riding the streets setting up and creating magic with a couple Vitamixes, freshly harvested greens, some fruit and ice and the joy of knowing that we were doing something simply good.

Sometimes when I transported myself back to those beginning days... Feed The 5000 and Alan, Patrick, Chris

Crosby, Paula, all of us trying to bring all this light and electricity to community, I was so lonely on that cold school bus that I would cry.

Now Paula was gone?

What a fool I was... trying to do something that seemed so simple, made so much sense and here I was about to be crushed emotionally, mentally. The current that was pulling so many of my comrades and allies down, was pulling me in.

For the first time I thought maybe people were right. Perhaps I was crazy to think that as an outsider, I would come here to this city with all of its rules, secret codes, corrupt politicians and super heavy war against the poor and think I was gonna change anything.

The dye had been cast long before I came to this place.

Maybe it was time for me to go... to leave Oakland.

There was one problem.

I'd done too much to turn around.

I'd made soul commitments... the boy with the gleaming eyes, he had not faded from my memory, but had morphed into the hundreds of young people I encountered at Juvenile Justice prisons, deep in the bowels of buildings where there were not only no abundantly flowing Green Smoothies, but also no sunlight... nothing living. His tender, excited eyes had morphed into and blended with the deferred hopes of the men at San Quentin... who recounted, during workshops, their greatest challenges as little ones before finding ways to escape... ways that led them to our circle and garden group at State Prison.

Though I felt like I was sleepwalking through quicksand, I knew I couldn't give up. As long as I had breath and energy, I couldn't give up. There was something supporting my staying on the ground here, despite the desperate nature of my circumstances and the things going on around me.

Besides that... where was I gonna go? This was my community now. I was being challenged and reprogrammed... and it was painful. I just had to keep moving with it, no matter how much it hurt.

And dude... did it hurt!

I now began to realize that Oakland was Ground Zero for Black folks, poor folks and children and elders moving through the world as part of this group. And once again, my mother's words came back to me...*Jim Crow...slavery.* At a very deep level, I understood what was happening and I knew...
in my heart, if I left without fulfilling my mission, I wouldn't be right with myself. I didn't know if I was gonna make it and prayed to God every day and night that I would, but I knew that I couldn't walk away.

There would be no facing myself in the mirror if I did..

HOW ARE YOU HEALING TODAY

I didn't feel well at all walking into the small, well lit chapel. I wasn't late, but the place was already packed.

It was Paula's memorial and not only her family was there, but there was an activist from every echelon of work in addition to throngs of folks from community that came because she was their friend and they felt truly loved by Paula. I sat in a pew near the front... and felt the intense sense of loss in the room.

She was gone.

The woman who held me tight and told me I'd never be an orphan as long as I had her... who called on me and checked for me when I was going through things and no one else seemed to notice or care... or could bear the weight of my sorrow.

Paula did.

She cared and loved all of us.

It was why the chapel was packed.

Well, when the person who had been organized to introduce the service did not appear, I waited a few beats and then got up to read from the program the minister placed in my hand.

I just remember the surrealness of seeing all those people looking back at me from the other side of the podium, the sadness in their faces and depth of loss. The only reason all those activists with so many issues and so much beef would ever assemble, I mean people who hadn't spoken in years... the only reason, I reminded myself, was because Paula must have been gone.

This is Paula's memorial, I reminded myself.

Paula is gone.

That's why I'm up here.

It almost knocked me off my feet, but I bit my tongue and did everything I could not to pass out... the grief seemed to hit me in one giant wave as I stood there with only the sound of my voice breaking the stillness of the palpable collective yearning for her beautiful spirit, her laughter, her love, her down to earth Christ Consciousness and humor... brought me back.

She was the one who stood beside us all, at one point or another, in public moments and more importantly in private moments that nobody else saw or cared about... stood by us in love... she was gone... what could we do?

Learn to love one another... the way she loved us, without judgment, like we were all her own.

Paula's spirit filled the room as person after person got up to speak her life, speak her support of them through her love and acceptance, through her humor and her knowledge of love as the greatest mechanism for change and her knowledge of justice as love in action... love walking. Folks got up and spoke through tears and oft with the support of translators to yield the same message: she loved us and she fought for justice!

Our guide had gone on, but she left us with many examples, and by the end of the day after being with her friends, her children, her grandchildren... I'd been healed.

The horizon, with children playing and drinking smoothies and organizing community in health and well-being, was clear and bright again.

Paula's Spirit had supported a clarity of consciousness for me and I was whole again, knowing that to succeed we had to, have to support one another's dreams, support one another's success... and to do this, we need to heal and ask one another everyday, How Are You Healing Today?

QUIET ON THE SET

As winter turned to spring I was still slugging it out, keeping the good fight. It was wearing me down, but my faith told me to steady my course. I didn't know what was going to happen next, so I pushed on. Sometimes all we can do is put one foot in front of the other and let the ground catch our step and our faith move us forward.

On May 11, 2017, I stood waiting for a city bus in front of Fazule and Sons Plumbing on the corner of Maple and Macarthur. I noticed, across the street, a groovy little artist space. It reminded me of Brooklyn or South Chicago, kind of rare for California.

As I stood waiting on the bus that seemed to be taking forever, I took out my phone and snapped a photograph of myself in the window. When the bus came, I kissed my girlfriend goodbye and got on. I was trying to divert my own attention from the heaviness in my heart, my sense of being overwhelmed. I pulled out my little journal and prayed for God to rescue me from so many of the things that were bringing me down in life and making me feel so tired and worn out... a troubled relationship that because of the housing market seemed impossible to leave behind; a place in my work where I felt in over my head and ineffective.

I sat on the bus and hoped, humbly for better days and the strength to persevere. As the bus made its way through the city, it was a sunny day, I felt how detached I felt from my surroundings and even though there were people laughing and talking and riding their bikes, it felt like a dark cloud was hovering over my world. I knew all I could do was hold on and things would get better.

A few days later I got a phone call from Derrick Mathis, a buddy of mine out in LA.

"Girl, you'll never believe what just happened. I just met a Casting Director, I'm sitting here in the dog park, letting NOLA run around and play and I over hear the woman, she says she looking for an artistic, original, kind of off the grid person....a freak, to do a commercial. Her name is Shannon. She's gonna call you in a few minutes. I just gave her your number. You pick up your phone girl. Don't not pick up your phone. Girl pick up your phone!"

I laughed at my buddy. He was... is... crazy.

The Casting Director did call.

Her name was indeed Shannon.

I told her about my life, my work, the housing situation and the school bus.

"I love that you actually live on a school bus. And you work in gardens and do smoothies for kids?! That's amazing. Can you shoot me a little 1 minute thing about yourself, on your Smartphone, so I can send it to the agency?"

Sure I could. Why not? It was weird, out of the blue, but I had nothing to lose. So I made the clip that afternoon when I got home, in front of my school bus with our dog Sausage poking her face out of the window. I talked about the smoothies, the street corners and the kids and the high schools... going into communities that had little if any living food, and blending smoothies to bring kids back into balance.

I heard back from Shannon pretty immediately. She made some suggestions, I followed her instructions and before I knew it, there were other Hollywood people calling about paperwork and asking me whether I could I travel to meet the Director.

Once again, Sure! Why not? I had nothing to lose. So I got together the only little outfit that I had really; a decent pair of jeans, a vest and a T-shirt that I bought at the Goodwill.

I fasted some toxins away... for a week or two, so I could look and feel my best, got on the train, and went to San Francisco.

Remember I said before that I worked with Derek Jeter's Foundation over at the Recreation Center in Harlem? Well, going to this interview felt very much like going to that interview. I felt like I was being guided by some unknown force that knew the outcome even though I didn't know what was going to happen... I knew it was gonna be good.

I had fun going to San Francisco. I don't really get out of Oakland much and it was a breath of fresh air. I felt like I'd been under water.

The interview was basically a room full of young, bright, Hollywood commercial folks, and a cheery Director from the UK.

We talked about what I could talk about forever, providing nutrition via smoothies for children. When he told me that his children weren't really crazy about Green Smoothies, I offered to come by his house and make them for him... everyone laughed.

We enjoyed the interview, and I left.

I got a call the next day or the day after saying that they wanted me to be a part of talent for their commercial.

They said there'd be lots of deadlines and a lot of Hollywood people calling freaking out with bunches of paperwork and background checks that needed to be handled. Pushing paper is not my forte. But I focused, got it together, and sent it to them.

The night before filming, early June, I'm laying in bed and a program about Nikola Tesla came on the TV.

Now I've seen just about every program about him, but this one told me something I did not know. He was obsessed with the number three. He said that the number 333 or nine holds the key to the universe. Once you've tapped into this and understand this, you pretty much hold the secret to the universe that we live in.

Everyone thought he was nuts.

That was interesting.

If everyone thought he was nuts and they thought I was nuts, I guess it gave us something in common.

The next day I made the drive out to Santa Cruz, beautiful,

beautiful, beautiful Santa Cruz, to misty, dewey gorgeous air, the ocean, that layer of mist that looms just above the surface of the water... the surfers... the seals... dolphins... the boardwalks.

I'd been so hunkered down with my work that I hadn't taken anytime lately to do anything fun. Now here I was for two nights in Santa Cruz checking into a beautiful hotel, stones throw from the beach.

As I checked in and surveyed the hotel actually called "Paradox," I was caught completely off guard when the guy checking me in gave me my room key "OK Miss Curry, you'll be in room 333."

I must have scrunched up my eyes. I asked him to repeat himself, "what did you just say what... what... what room?"

"333... is that all right Miss Curry... or would you like another room?"

"No," I said "That's absolutely fabulous, 333 is perfect."

As I made my way to the room, I had that feeling that I have every so often. It's difficult to explain, but I'll try, it's like every piece of reality that has been carefully constructed around me has fallen away and the only thing that I'm standing in is a bubble of magic. It's as if the commercial out of the blue... out of nowhere wasn't enough, now I will check into a room with the number 333, which only last night I hear holds the keys to unlocking the secrets of the universe.

The universe is speaking very loudly to me in this moment. I was all ears, heart and soul. "This is the beginning of the end of this movie... the end of the dark days... my prayers answered," I say to myself as I run the key against the door and open into room 333.

That night I sat down thinking about Tesla, thinking about the Green Smoothies, seeing that horizon again... clearly before my eyes, children happy healthy preparing their own Green Smoothies and enjoying the abundance of the Earth as God intends for us to enjoy... How Are You Healing Today? Part of everyone's consciousness asking the question and answering the question through diligent patience and sustainable practices.

The vision appeared before me so clearly that I took a pen and my little journal, the same one with my scribbled prayer at the bus stop on May 11 and I wrote something that will stand with me forever.

This I know was a gift from Nikola. It is a gift from Paula. It is a gift from my mother and the gift from my father.

I'll put it here so you can see it.

It is not us
But the Energy that roils
Through our bodies
our Soul,
igniting,
animating our potential
our ideas
our creativity
our love
this is all love,
this Electricity
a gift
a battery
from our maker
Nature is the core of our existence of our ability
to be creative
and participate
as particles of central organizing that we are
without this love
moving through us
we are nothing.

I went to sleep and dreamt about that horizon, and in the morning got a phone call from someone I hadn't talked to in a very long time. She was the caretaker for the spot on MacArthur, the place I'd stood in front of, where I photographed myself in the window while I waited on the city bus that day, May 11.

She asked me whether I would like to move in. I was so shocked, I couldn't quite wrap my mind around what was happening.

I was beyond shocked. "You can open your smoothie shop," she said "it's a live workspace... are you still in your bus?"

I told her yes indeed I was.

"Well put your paperwork in with this place, it's perfect for you."

With that the car arrived to take us to the set. My mind and my heart were busy.

WOW!!!!

The Universe was talking, that's all I could think. It was as if a chariot had arrived, just pulled up and pulled me out and away from the dismal circumstances that felt like they were crushing me.

When we arrived at the set it was probably the most beautiful thing I'd seen in a long time.

The commercial was to be filmed at a tulip farm. There were millions and millions and millions of tulips... seas of tulips everywhere. After being prepped and pampered, fooded and powdered... hair and make-up and waiting my turn in the Winnebago with the make-up girls and producer who is bouncing around and finally my name came up and I was summonsed.

I went and stood in front of the biggest camera I'd ever seen in my life, surrounded by the tulips and the soft bright lights held in place by a crew of seven or eight technicians.

When the Director asked me how I felt being there, all I could hear after he yelled "quiet on the set" was the sound of those beautiful tulips. The sound of all the beautiful nature around me, the purity of it so intense, "it's so beautiful, can't you hear them talking to us?" If they hadn't spent all that time on my hair and make-up I would have cried tears of joy, I enjoyed the silence for as long as I could, and some part of me, that same part of me that stood at the podium in front of all of those faces and all those people with that sadness when we came together to say goodbye to Paula, the same thing in me that goes completely at ease and grounds me, went completely at ease.

The Director and I chatted about smoothies and children and nutrition in the non-GMO vitamin Sundown Naturals created. We laughed in the field of flowers and for a while I was there on that horizon, really calling it in and happy to share about it.

It was fun, and before I knew, it was over.

I spent that night in the hotel and relished the privilege of knowing that my thoughts and my actions were making up the world I wanted to live in.

I had some beautiful dreams that night, and in addition to a heck of a story, I also had something else I didn't have before... my faith restored. I had recovered the knowledge that God heard me, that I hadn't been forgotten.

THE TABLE

I asked Annie and James to come meet me at the place. It was a Saturday afternoon and the sun was shining. I'd gotten the keys from my new landlord the day before. We'd sat in a cafe in Santa Cruz and I signed the lease. "I love the work you're doing. We need more people like you in the world. You know I got twenty five calls for that place the first hour I had the sign in the window and on paper you don't look like much, your credit needs a lot of help, but I love the work you're doing and I have a feeling you won't let me down. I'll never raise your rent and I'll support your work in any way I can."

The whole thing was surreal.

I felt my mother and Paula's imprint on the whole thing. I mean a month after I'd stood at the bus stop in front of Fazule and Sons Plumbing and taken that picture of myself in the window... said that prayer... here I was sitting with this beautiful, bright eyed, intelligent woman (a writer too!) the landlord... signing a lease.

With the money I'd made from the commercial and a settlement from an illegal eviction, my lawyer Mark Hooshmond and his attorneys had helped me win, I was able to come up with the money—first and last and the first few months of rent at what I thought we should call The Electric Smoothie Lab.

I opened the door and walked in with Annie and James, two friends of mine and the community who truly understood the connection between eradicating children's health disparities, the prison industrial complex and Green Smoothies.

We all stood in the space looked at the giant windows and hardwood floors together and Annie smiled and gave me a huge hug, "OH KELLY! I'm so happy and excited for you! Now you can do all the things you've been talking about."

"This is dope!" James said, "This place is amazing." They took a photo of me in the window, this time I was standing inside... under the bright sunlight and after they left I closed the doors and stood alone in the large open, sunny space. Everything had happened so fast that I had a hard time wrapping my mind around it. I mean, I was still living on my bus. I loved my bus. People asked me why and I just felt like I had to give myself time to understand what had happened... and what was happening. Since I didn't organize it, plan it and make it happen in all the ways we humans think we have to plan and organize things, really I was quite shocked and wanted to treat the opportunity as pristinely as it was...which meant that I had to let it unfold the way God intended.

I really didn't want to get in the way.

So even though it was a live-work space, and I was paying rent, I didn't move in. I parked my bus outside and lived in it.

I made smoothies there every morning, had a launch gathering, but somehow, after everything I'd been through, I was afraid to commit.

Can you believe it?

Part of me was so crushed and so sad and so devastated... traumatized I guess... from the year before and still processing it all...what I'd been through, what I'd seen and what had happened, that I wasn't sure if I wanted to stay in Oakland at all. God stepping in with the commercial and the settlement and the The Electric Lab, just ramped up the pressure. If I was gonna leave Oakland, take a pass and chalk it up to a weird adventure, this would be the time... otherwise I'd be all in and there'd be no turning back.

"You're talkin' leavin' again?" A good friend of mine said... "You got the LAB, now you wanna leave?"

The idea of planning anything else besides the next step— and even that was a lot—exhausted me. I was spun out. Overexposed and mourning the loss of so much. But at the same time, I was pushing myself to make this thing happen, even though I knew in my heart, that since I hadn't "made it happen" it was in my eyes a mystical act. I knew that I couldn't push anything. I accepted that I needed time off to recalibrate and let my human body and mind catch up to what had started to feel like a magical, divine journey.

Even though I wanted to, I didn't stay at the Lab.

Something in me wouldn't give the green light.

I guess I still hadn't committed to yielding my spirit to renewing the fight of bringing the one Green Smoothie a day to the children, the ones most in need and suffering from food insecurity. It had almost killed me, really, did I wanna jump back in?

Then one day, when I got to the Lab to set up to do Smoothies and make deliveries, I noticed a table sitting on the corner, leaned up against the side of my door. People were always leaving things... couches, neatly folded blankets... vases... little odds and ends on that corner, maybe as a "one man's trash another man's treasure" type offering.

I looked at it, it was nice enough, good, solid, old wooden dining room or kitchen table. The four legs were wrapped up together neatly. I knew if I brought it in and set it up, it would mean that I was staying. Since I wasn't sure yet... in my heart... I left it there and went about my chores and tasks for the morning. In emotional torment... cleaning the Lab, moving things around... going through the motions really, cuz if your heart isn't in something, what's the use... and I knew it and I hated it. But still I did the things that I believed I should be doing and just the same, after a long day at the Lab, went home around 1 am or so.

When I came back the next morning I noticed that the table was still there. No one had claimed it. Pity. Nice table. It was still propped in the same position, "kitty corner" as my mom would say, against the side of the building. Once again I went about my daily chores, faking moves and doing all the things I thought I should... my heart someplace else and my healing taking its time.

On the third day... I drove up the block, the sun streaming into the road and something radiant hit my eye as soon as I glanced towards my place. The table was still there, but this morning, even though it was still propped kitty corner, in the same position it was in when I saw it three four days ago, this morning it had a portrait on it.

It was a graffiti breakdown of a beautiful, full lipped sister with giant hoop earrings, arched eyebrows and an expression in her eyes that conveyed the songs of all your dreams, thoughts, prayers, heartbreaks, illusions, fantasies and get up again and make it so's. It was a work in black with a purple outline...my mother's favorite color.

I'll never forget the feeling my heart... my Soul stirring for the first time in months... my passion igniting to movement and energy...grabbing the portrait off the street corner, placing it in the light, knowing in my heart that it was a sign from my beloved guide. My mother. Telling me that if I chose to stay in Oakland and organize the nutrition for the children... that I would be guided, guarded and my mission delivered.

She would be with me... she'd been with me the whole time.

I photographed the portrait, which must have been painted in the wee hours of the morning, since I'd left the lab at around 1 am just that morning and returned at 7:30 am. I sent the photo to my aunt Kathy in Kansas City, my buddy Haleh, Monika in NYC, Stephanie in SC and a few other folks who knew me, my mother, my dreams and my story.

Within a few seconds I received responses from the several parts of the US via text.."OMG DUDE...That's your mom!" What is she trying to tell you?

INSIDE THE GREEN SMOOTHIE

Because greens are the flowers of the earth, the children of the amazing communication between earth and sun and rain and air—a perfect, powerful punch of chlorophyll and more vitamins and minerals than you can believe or imagine—putting them in your body everyday is going to change you at a cellular level and change the way you relate to the world and to yourself. If you let it.

Take one single kale leaf, put it under water and watch it glow. There is magic in there.

Imagine all of that magic, all of that energy, comprised from millions and millions of years of communication between the stars and the minerals of our Mother Earth, including fossils and stardust and the Sun and participation of rain UNDOING what my Grandmama Nelly would call the foolishness of "fast food," commercial meat and dairy, and what we know of as "snacks."

Imagine what all of this ancient information pulled together, miraculously, into a leaf of kale or spinach or beet green or purple tree collard is doing as it works its way through your colon, scrubs your intestines and cleanses years and years and years of solid waste impacted into the inner pockets of parts of the inner lining of your belly that is craving and yearning to breathe again.

As a result of making Green Smoothies everyday for clients and school children and community folks at schools, elder centers and community demonstrations, I am always dealing with greens in my hands, whether I'm harvesting or going through greens at the Food Mill or making smoothies and tasting them and drinking them all day myself.

What I've noticed is the changes in my energy levels, the shifts in my palette and the depth of vitality that I experience, it's deep, lasting and quite frankly astounding.

The regimen has changed my way of being in the world.

I'm much calmer, a lot more mellow and have more

patience to think things through and be in relationship with my work, my family and friends in a way that is positive, patient and meaningful. My outlook about the things happening on a global level, (daunting and insurmountable as they appear a times) is positive and clear. I'm a better organizer and community person. I drink less alcohol, even though I still LOVE my California Reds, it's simply something I enjoy to enjoy in moderation and that is truly a gift.

This is the thing though—I'm not working at any of it. Since I began drinking Green Smoothies everyday as a part of my work, I simply crave the light and energy and availability of healing I receive from the electricity of the greens and the beauty of the variety of fruits and herbs that I blend and pour into the cup.

The fact that I can share it all at a time when so many folks who are ailing and suffering from food related illnesses is wonderful. The fact that everyone who heals from it, agrees with me that children and community who are shut off from it, need it, is an even greater bonus.

Today, the most vulnerable, the little boy on the street corner, his family and others nationwide are suffering tyrannies that all of us, if engaged, can support in alleviating... but we gotta have the strength.

All smoothies are not created equal

If you're organizing your little ones away from refined sugar and moving towards Green Smoothies, start with spinach, plenty of sweet herbs like basil and pineapple sage and their favorite fruits. Sooner than later you'll be able to start using Kale and Collards and other greens. You can also freeze Green Smoothies into popsicles and ice cubes.

Remember to use ripe bananas, preferably lightly to heavily spotted. They are the best because they are less starchy and they've started the process of digestion--the starch has moved to sugar already and is immediately available. If you are diabetic use less of the sweet fruits like banana and use more apple, lemon, and berries.

Your job is to make it taste the way you like it. So feel free to experiment with the amounts I have listed here. Here's some recipes to get us back in the game.

Easy Good Summer Smoothie
1-2 cups of Spinach
1 whole ripe Banana
½ cup of Strawberries
Handful of Mint
Cup and Half of Spring Water

Easy Green Good Circulation Smoothie
1-2 cups of Spinach
1 whole ripe Banana
½ cup of Strawberries
Handful of Mint
Teaspoon of Turmeric
½ teaspoon shredded Ginger
1 ½ cup Spring Water

Super Scrub Smoothie
3-4 Kale leaves
2-3 Collards leaves
Tablespoon Chia Seeds
½ cup Blueberries
1 Apple
1 Mango
1 whole ripe Banana
1-2 cups Spring Water

Please be creative, have fun, experiment with your Smoothies and remember, keep it green, at least once a day.

ABOUT THE AUTHOR

Kelly Curry is an author, publisher and social justice activist. She brings over 20 years of frontline, on the ground support of lower income communities of color through her development of life enhancing, ground shifting programs that promote health, well being and love. A veteran of public and private foundation work in New York City, Kelly was influential in ushering in change around public children's after-school programming at the city level, which included development and successful operation of a living arts program for NYC Parks and Recreation Center in Harlem. Through this program, Kelly worked with community kids to plant Harlem's first children's gardens. Kelly continued this trajectory by delivering a living arts program to the children of farm workers and homeless children in Southern California via The Living Love Foundation, where she acted as Director of Programming and Development. Kelly is currently focused on engaging committed, creative, sustainable change around food access for the citizens of East and West Oakland. She does this work in partnership with Planting Justice via How Are You Healing Today which hosts The Electric Smoothie Lab Apothecary.

ABOUT THE COVER ARTIST

Annie Banks is an organizer/artist in Berkeley, California, on Ohlone territories. Annie is an active member of the California Coalition for Women Prisoners and the Anti Police-Terror Project and has been a printmaker since high school. "The role of cultural workers is important in our movements for justice." For more information: www.anniebanks.net.

www.ingramcontent.com/pod-product-compliance
Lightning Source LLC
Chambersburg PA
CBHW022110160426
43198CB00008B/421